# SUGAR RESET

## :your 21-day Transformation

Dr.Maggie W Engler

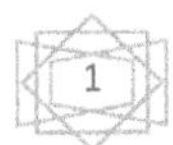

All right reserved. No part of this publication may be
reproduced, distributed, or
transmitted in any form or by any means, including
photocopying,recording,or
other electronic or mechanical method, without the prior
written permission of the
publisher, except in the case of brief quotations embodied
in critical review and
certain other non-commercial uses permitted by copyright
law.
Copyright © Dr. Maggie W Engler , 2023.

In its many forms, sugar has ingrained itself into the fundamental fabric of our existence. It is a persistent companion, a nagging temptation, and frequently a deceiving one. We will delve deeply into the alluring world of sugar in this first chapter of "Sugar Reset: Your 21-Day Transformation," revealing its hidden facets and explaining why it is so difficult to escape its sweet hold.

**Sugar's Seductive Power**
Sugar has had a hypnotic effect on our senses ever since we first tasted it as infants. Its sweetness mesmerizes our taste buds and sets off a chain reaction of delightful feelings in our bodies. Our lifetime connection with sugar is built on this need for instant fulfillment.

Sugar has changed over time from being a rare treat to being a common ingredient in our meals. It can also be found in common foods like ketchup, bread, and even what appears to be nutritious yogurt. It is not only present in obvious sources like sweets and soda. This ubiquitous nature makes it a strong foe in our fight for greater health.

**The Sugar Spectrum**
We must first acknowledge that sugar comes in a variety of forms to fully comprehend its effects. Sugars are not all made equal. The two main kinds are sugars that exist naturally and sugars that are added.

Sugars That Occur Naturally: These sugars are a natural component of some foods, including dairy, vegetables, and fruits. They contain a variety of important nutrients, including fiber, vitamins, and minerals, which slow down their absorption and lessen any adverse effects they may have on the body.

**Additional Sugars:** These are the sugars that food producers include in their products as they process or prepare them. They go by a variety of names, including sucrose, agave nectar, and high fructose corn syrup. Added sugars provide worthless calories that are devoid of any substantial nutrition. Herein lays the sweet trap's real catch.

**The Sweet Deception**
Sugar's capacity to take on many names makes it one of the most ingenious tricks in the book. Even the most health-conscious people find it tough to recognize and stay away from added sugars due to the abundance of these aliases on food labels. Just a few of the guises it dons are as follows:

High-fructose corn syrup (HFCS): HFCS is a highly processed sugar that is frequently included in processed foods and sweetened beverages. It can seriously mess with our metabolism.

- Sugar (Sucrose) This is regular table sugar, which is frequently used in baking and beverage sweetening. Even while it may appear benign, excessive use can nonetheless be a source of added sugars.

- Agave nectar Agave nectar is marketed as a natural sweetener, although this is deceptive. It contains a lot of fructose, which, when ingested in excess, can harm the body.

- Evaporated Cane Juice Doesn't this sound like a good idea? Sadly, it's just another way of saying "sugar."

It is difficult for people to understand the degree of their sugar consumption since the sugar business has successfully dispersed its numerous forms throughout the ingredient lists of processed foods.

## The Reaction of the Brain

Understanding sugar's tricks involves more than just being aware of what it hides; it also entails being aware of how it alters our minds. In the reward areas of the brain, sugar, especially in the form of high-fructose corn syrup, causes dopamine release.

A neurotransmitter linked to reward and pleasure is dopamine. Dopamine is released in our brains in large amounts when we eat sugar, which makes us feel good and satisfied. This response is comparable to what happens when addictive substances, like narcotics, are consumed.

As a result, our brains start to want that delightful experience, which motivates us to consume more sugar. This urge may spiral into an unending cycle, resulting in overeating and the ensuing health issues.

**The Insulin Rollercoaster**

Sugar has a significant impact on our bodies in addition to the brain, particularly on blood sugar levels and insulin synthesis.

Our blood sugar levels rise when we eat or drink something sugary. The pancreas responds by releasing insulin to control this surge in sugar. The main function of insulin is to transport sugar into our cells for use as fuel or storage.

However, this system might get overworked if we consistently overfeed our bodies with sugar.

Cells that have developed insulin resistance in the body no longer react to insulin as effectively. This syndrome, which increases the risk of weight gain and cardiovascular disease, is a precursor to type 2 diabetes.

The Sweet Seduction
The capacity of sugar to creep into our lives without our knowledge is arguably one of its most cunning strategies. Let's think about a few instances where sugar inadvertently enters our diets:

**Coffee in the morning**
You might go to your preferred coffee shop for a latte as part of your seemingly innocent morning routine. What you may not know is that whipped cream toppings and flavored syrups can significantly increase the quantity of sugar you consume each day.

**"Healthy" Snacks**
You decide to eat better options, so you buy a yogurt or granola bar from the shop. These goods frequently present themselves as wholesome choices. A brief scan of the label reveals hidden additional sugars, though.

Menu at Restaurant
When eating out with pals, you decide on a salad that sounds delicious. You might not be aware that the dressing may include more sugar than you might anticipate. Even restaurants' savory food can be loaded with extra sweets.

**Social Get-togethers**
When you go to a birthday party or family reunion, sweets

are a given. It's simple to overindulge in sweet treats on these occasions without even realizing it.

Sugar's alluring allure lurks in everyday decisions and circumstances. It is especially difficult to escape its hold because of its ubiquity.

## The Relation Between Sugar and Health

We must examine sugar's significant influence on our health to properly appreciate the relevance of comprehending its deceitful methods. The long and concerning list of health problems linked to high sugar consumption includes:

- **Obesity:** The link between sugar and weight growth is well established. Its extra caloric content can easily tip the scales in favor of obesity, which is connected to several illnesses like heart disease, diabetes, and several malignancies.
- **Diabetes type 2:** Consuming too much sugar can cause insulin resistance, which is a precursor to type 2 diabetes. This can eventually lead to high blood sugar levels and the requirement for medication to treat the illness.
- **Heart Condition:** By encouraging inflammation, raising blood pressure, and causing high triglyceride levels, a high-sugar diet can raise the risk of heart disease.
- **Dental Issues:** The main cause of tooth decay and cavities is sugar. Our oral bacteria feed on sugar and produce acids that destroy tooth enamel.
- Fat Liver Disorder: Consuming too much sugar, particularly fructose, can cause non-alcoholic fatty

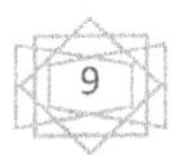

liver disease (NAFLD), which can develop into more serious liver issues.

- Mental Health Recent studies point to a link between excessive sugar consumption and mental health problems like sadness and anxiety. Consuming sugar can cause blood sugar spikes and crashes that can impact mood and general well-being.

Knowing how sugar tricks your body is more than just a nutrition exercise; it's an essential step in ensuring your long-term health and well-being. The delicious trap is real, but you can escape it with knowledge and willpower.

## Grasp.

The chapters that follow will go into greater detail on the science underlying sugar's impacts, look at realistic tactics for cutting back, and take you on a transforming 21-day journey that will give you the power to take charge of your health and your life. With this knowledge in hand, you're now prepared to take the first step on the road to sugar liberation.

## Chapter 2.
### Unmasking Sugar: The Diet's Hidden Culprits

Thank you for visiting Chapter 2 of "Sugar Reset: Your 21-Day Transformation." We will go on a journey of discovery as we expose the covert sources of sugar in your diet in this chapter. It's important to realize that sugar may be sneaky, hiding in plain sight within seemingly benign foods and drinks. You will get the knowledge necessary to make knowledgeable decisions and take control of your sugar intake by exposing these hidden sources of sugar.

## Sugar's Cunning Nature

Sugar sneakily makes its way into our meals. Although we may be careful to avoid sugary snacks and sweets, they frequently sneak into our meals through unforeseen channels. The outcome? Unknowingly, we consume more sugar than we realize, which can lead to a variety of health problems, such as heart disease and weight gain.

We must first comprehend the various shapes that sugar might take to reveal it:

**Natural Sugars**
Whole foods like fruits and dairy products naturally contain sugar. These sugars are healthier options because they contain fiber and important minerals that decrease the absorption of sugar.

**Added Sugars**
What we need to watch out for are added sugars. These are sugars that are added to meals and drinks while they are being processed or prepared. They give off inert calories and may cause health issues.

Let's investigate some of the diet's covert sources of added sugar now:

**Sweetened Drinks**

Sugary drinks like soda, fruit juices, and energy drinks are among the major sources of added sugar. These beverages might have a high sugar content without making you feel full, which can result in consuming too many calories.

**Step into Action:** Water, herbal tea, or unsweetened alternatives should be used in place of sweetened drinks. Slices of citrus fruit or herbs can be used to flavor water.

## Cereals for Breakfast

Even those promoted as healthy selections, many morning cereals might include a lot of added sugar. Some well-known cereals have as much sugar in them as candy bars.

**Step into Action:** Choose low-sugar, whole-grain cereals or oatmeal that has been sprinkled with cinnamon and topped with fresh fruit.

- **Yogurts**
  Yogurts with flavors, especially those that have fruit at the bottom, can be sugar bombs. Yogurt includes lactose, which naturally contains sugars, but added sweets frequently overpower them.

**Step into Action:** Make your fresh fruit additions or add a splash of honey for natural sweetness to plain, unsweetened yogurt.

- **Condiments and Sauces:** Ketchup, barbeque sauce, and salad dressings can all contain unexpected amounts of sugar. Your meals are sweetened without you even recognizing it.

**Step into Action:** Pay close attention to the labels and choose condiments without added sugars, or prepare your own at home using better products.

- **Energy and granola bars:** Granola and energy bars that are touted as healthy food sometimes include a ton of extra sugar. They are frequently promoted as time-saving solutions for busy people, but they can also lead to sugar excess.

**Step into Action:** Pick bars that have a small amount of sugar added, or even better, create your own at home using complete foods like oats, almonds, and dried fruits.

- **Packaged Foods:** Crackers, chips, and even savory snacks can have hidden sugars in them. These sugars make food taste better and promote intake.

**Step into Action:** To avoid sneaky sugars, choose whole-food snacks like hummus and raw vegetables or a handful of unsalted nuts.

- **Quick Oatmeal**
  Although handy, pre-packaged flavored oatmeal packets frequently have additional sugars added to improve flavor.

**Step into Action:** Pick plain oats and customize them with your favorite toppings, such as fresh fruit, nuts, and honey or maple syrup.

Food Label Decoding Your superpower in the fight against hidden sugar is reading food labels. Pay attention to the ingredient list because sugars might be found there under a variety of names, including

**High Fructose Corn Syrup**
**Sucrose**
**Agave Nectar**
**Fruit Juice Concentrate**
**Cane Sugar**
**Honey**
**Molasses**
**Dextrose**
**Malt Syrup, among others**

Be watchful and ask questions about the product's sugar content if you notice these or similar terms prominently included in the ingredient list.

## The 21-Day Transformation and Hidden Sugar

A crucial part of your journey will be identifying and exposing hidden sugar as you start your 21-day makeover. Making informed decisions regarding common foods and drinks is just as important as avoiding overtly sweet delicacies.

**To successfully find hidden sugar**

Read all labels Make it a routine to read food labels carefully for added sugars. Look for
sugar aliases in the ingredient list with particular attention.

- Opt for entire foods: Choosing whole, unprocessed foods will reduce the likelihood that they contain hidden sugars. These consist of whole grains, lean proteins, fresh fruits and vegetables, and fruits.

- Cook meals at home: When you prepare meals at home, you have complete control over the components. You can pick healthier options and change the sweetness to your preference.
- Be mindful: Take time to appreciate the tastes of your food and drink. Your taste buds might adapt over time to enjoy less sweetness.
- Learn more about: Be aware of how much sugar is present in popular meals and beverages. Your best line of protection against hidden sugar is knowledge.

Keep in mind that your 21-day change is about developing long-lasting habits that support health and well-being, not merely momentarily reducing your sugar intake. You're taking a big step toward accomplishing your sugar control goals and embracing a healthier, more active lifestyle by exposing hidden sugar and making thoughtful decisions.

## Chapter 3:
### Taming Your Sugar Demons: Craving Control

Thank you for visiting Chapter 3 of "Sugar Reset: Your 21-Day Transformation." We examine one of the most important obstacles on your path to sugar control in this chapter: cravings. We'll look at the psychological underpinnings of sugar cravings, the science behind them, and techniques to help you recover control over your cravings for indulgent sweets.

## Sugar Cravings: The Science

Cravings have a scientific foundation established in biology and brain chemistry and are not just random whims. Understanding the mechanisms underlying these desires is essential if you want to learn how to conquer your sugar demons.

**The pleasure principle and dopamine**

Dopamine, a neurotransmitter linked to reward and pleasure, is at the root of sugar cravings. Dopamine is released into the body when you eat sugary foods, giving you a pleasurable feeling. This internal mechanism of reinforcement increases the desire for sugar.

**Rollercoaster for Blood Sugar**

Excessive sugar consumption produces sharp blood sugar increases followed by crashes. Your body seeks rapid sources of energy, frequently in the form of sugar, when your blood sugar levels fall. This rollercoaster impact may cause cravings, which would keep the cycle going.

**Ghrelin and leptin**

Leptin and ghrelin are two hormones that regulate hunger and satiety. The "hunger hormone," ghrelin, stimulates appetite while leptin conveys a sense of fullness. These hormone disruptions may cause increased appetites, especially for sweet foods.

**Mental Contributors to Sugar Cravings**
Sugar cravings are impacted by psychological and emotional variables in addition to physiological ones. Let's investigate the psychological causes of sugar cravings:

**Emotional eating**
Emotional eating frequently results from emotional triggers such as stress, boredom, worry, and melancholy. Sugary foods are seductive options during emotional situations since they can calm and relieve bad emotions.

1. **Action Step**: Develop alternate coping strategies, such as deep breathing exercises, meditation, or taking up an activity you enjoy, to help you deal with stress and emotions.

**Rewards Program**
Many of us have been socialized from an early age to equate sweets with festivities and rewards. Even as adults, these memories continue to fuel our appetites for pleasure or a sense of accomplishment.

2. **Step into Action:** Reconsider your system of rewards and find healthier ways to reward yourself. Think about giving yourself a spa day, a new book, or a stroll around the park as a reward.

**Regular Eating**
Repetitive actions can develop into habits, and regularly indulging in sugary foods and drinks can become a daily

routine that is difficult to quit. These behaviors may result in routinely induced cravings.

3. **Step into Action:** Determine your ingrained eating habits and replace them with more wholesome ones. Switch to nutrient-rich alternatives like fresh fruit or almonds in favor of sugary snacks.

## Environment-Related Triggers

Sugary temptations can be abundant in our environment. Cravings may be triggered by the sight, smell, or proximity of sweet foods. Environmental triggers can come from social events, ads, and even the design of grocery stores.

4. **Step into Action:** Reduce your exposure to situations that make you need sugar. Avoid having sugary snacks around the house, and limit your travel to places where there is a lot of temptation.

## Methods for Controlling Sugar Cravings

We can better manage our sugar cravings now that we are aware of the science and psychology involved.

## Eating Mindfully:

The ability to eat mindfully can help you beat your sugar cravings. It entails focusing intently on the sensory aspects of eating, appreciating each bite, and being in the present.

5. ***Step into Action***: By eating slowly, appreciating the flavors, and avoiding distractions like phones or TVs, you can practice mindful eating. This makes it easier for you to recognize hunger and fullness cues.

## Balanced Meals

Blood sugar levels can be stabilized by eating balanced meals that contain protein, good fats, and fiber-rich carbohydrates. Energy dips that cause a desire for sugary snacks are avoided by eating balanced meals.

Prioritize nutritious, well-balanced meals to maintain a constant level of energy throughout the day.

**Water intake**

 keeping hydrated is essential for controlling cravings. Sometimes people confuse hunger with thirst, which causes them to eat needless snacks.

Drink a lot of water throughout the day as an action step. Without using additional sugar, taste can be added to herbal teas and infused waters.

**Nutritious Snacks**

Having a variety of wholesome, ready-to-eat snacks on hand will help you avoid making rash decisions. Healthy between-meal snacks, such as diced veggies and hummus, Greek yogurt, berries, or a handful of mixed nuts, might quell your appetite.

6. *Action Step:* To prevent reaching for sugary foods, prepare nutritious snacks in advance and keep them close at hand.

**Stress management**

Techniques for managing stress well can lessen the need to eat sugar to feel better. Stress-relieving techniques include regular exercise, meditation, deep breathing exercises, and asking friends or a therapist for help.

Develop healthy coping strategies to manage stress without turning to sugary treats by identifying your stressors.

### Rest and Sleep

A lack of sleep and weariness can make sugar cravings worse by interfering with the hormones that control hunger and fullness. Put rest and good sleep first as part of your plan to manage your blood sugar.

7. *Action Step:* To enhance the quality of your sleep, adopt a calming nighttime routine and stick to a regular sleep schedule.

### Establishing a Support Network

With the help of others, taming your sugar demons is frequently much simpler. Tell your loved ones, a support group, or your friends about your objectives and difficulties. Having a network of people who are familiar with your journey can offer support and accountability.

### Honor Your Successes

It's a major accomplishment every time you successfully withstand a sugar craving or make a deliberate decision. Enjoy these wins as they come along. Treat yourself to non-food rewards that support your objectives to acknowledge your progress and strengthen your resolve to manage your sugar intake.

### Summary

Remember that controlling your sugar cravings is a journey rather than a quick fix as you move on with your 21-day makeover. It calls for dedication, introspection, and a readiness to look into the causes of your urges. Applying the techniques described in this chapter will give you the tools you need to recover control over your sugar cravings and lay the groundwork for long-term sugar control and general well-being. Accept the process, practice mindfulness, and make craving management a key component of your sugar reset journey.

## Sneaky Sugars: Using the Aisles of the Grocery Store

Thank you for visiting Chapter 4 of "Sugar Reset: Your 21-Day Transformation." We'll delve into the center of your sugar control quest in this chapter: the grocery store. You can find some of the sneakiest sources of added sugars here, among the busy aisles and vibrant displays. You'll discover how to maneuver these aisles like a pro and make healthier decisions that support your sugar reset goals armed with information and a calculated strategy.

**Sugar Landscape in a Grocery Store**

When trying to cut back on your sugar intake, navigating the grocery store can be challenging. A surprising number of ostensibly healthy goods and pantry staples include added sugars. Let's examine the layout of the grocery shop and look for potential sugar traps to successfully address this challenge:

**Produce Section**
Your first trip should be to the produce aisle, which is a paradise for healthy, low-sugar items. You can build your diet around this variety of fresh fruits and veggies if you're trying to cut back on sugar. Fruits have inherent sweetness without additional sugars including berries, apples, and citrus.

8. ***Step into Action***: Put a colorful assortment of fresh food in your shopping cart. These nutrient-dense foods will not only satiate your palate but also supply fiber and other vitamins.

**Perimeter Alleys**
Typically, fresh, natural goods like dairy, meats, and shellfish are located around the store's perimeter. Although

it's important to read labels on items like flavored yogurt and marinated meats, these categories are less likely to have added sugars.

9. ***Step into Action***: Concentrate on purchasing whole, unadulterated foods from the outside aisles. To prevent hidden sugars, choose plain dairy products and unseasoned meats and fish.

Center Aisles

Sugar-conscious customers may find the central aisles of the grocery store to be a dangerous area. Here you'll find a lot of packaged and processed goods as well as some of the sneakiest sources of added sugars.

We'll approach the middle aisles category by category to properly navigate them:

**Cereals for Breakfast**

Cereals for breakfast may include sugar landmines. Even foods that are promoted as healthful can have too much-added sugar. Pay great attention to the ingredient and nutrition labels.

10. ***Step into Action***: Choose low-sugar, whole-grain cereals, or think about making your oatmeal and seasoning it with fruit and spices.

**Seasonings**

Hidden sugars can be found in condiments including ketchup, barbecue sauce, and salad dressings. Look for items without added sugars on the label or make your own at home.

11. *Action Step:* Pick condiments with low sugar content or prepare your own at home with better ingredients.

## Snack Foods

To improve flavor, additional sugars are frequently used in chips, crackers, and salty snacks. Although appealing, these snacks might lead to excessive sugar consumption.

12. *Step into Action:* When choosing snacks, look for low- or no-added-sugar options. Think about substituting whole-food snacks like raw nuts or diced veggies for processed snack options.

## Toppings and soups

For flavor, sugar is frequently added to sauces and soups. Pay close attention to labels and think about making more meals from home to keep an eye on the components.

13. *Step into Action:* Choose sauces and soups without added sweeteners or try making your own using natural ingredients.

## Prepared Food

Although convenient, frozen and packaged meals may contain a lot of hidden sugars. Examine labels carefully and select products with the fewest added sugars.

14. *Step into Action*: Reduce your dependency on prepackaged meals, and when you do, choose items with less sugar.

## Beverages

Some of the worst offenders in the center aisles are drinks with added sugar. Energy drinks, sodas, and fruit juices can all contribute to overindulging in sugar without making you feel full.

15. ***Action Step:*** Switch to water, herbal tea, or other unsweetened liquids in place of sugary ones. Fruit juices should be avoided because they sometimes contain a lot of added sugar.



Your best tool in the grocery store is to become an expert label reader. Here's how to effectively interpret food labels:

**Verify the Ingredients**

 Your main information source is the list of ingredients. Look for added sugars, which can be concealed by several names, including:

High Fructose Corn Syrup
Sucrose
Agave Nectar
Fruit Juice Concentrate
Cane Sugar
Honey
Molasses
Dextrose
Malt Syrup among others

Be cautious and steer clear of products that use these or similar terms frequently in the ingredient list.

16. ***Action Step:*** Become familiar with sugar aliases and give preference to goods with fewer added sugars.



The sugar amount of a product can be learned from the Nutrition Facts label. The "Total Sugars" line, which contains both natural and added sugars, deserves special attention. Compare the amount to the "Added Sugars" line, which was added to the label to distinguish between the two, to determine the added sugar quantity.

Step into Action: Look for items with less added and total sugar. Pick foods and drinks that mostly include natural sources of sugar, such as fruits or dairy.

Smart Grocery Purchasing
Now that you are proficient in reading labels, let's look at some tips for a successful sugar-free supermarket shopping trip:

Be Prepared
Make a list of healthy foods, such as fresh produce, lean proteins, whole grains, and other products, before you go shopping. Making a plan will aid in maintaining focus and preventing rash purchases.

Action Step: Based on your program, plan your meals for the upcoming week and make a shopping list.

Shop the Periphery
Fresh, unprocessed items are often kept at the store's perimeter, as was already mentioned. Start your shopping there and stock up on nutrient-dense foods.

Organize your shopping so that the produce, dairy, meat, and seafood areas come first.

Reduce purchases made in the center aisle
Keep to your shopping list as you make your way through the center aisles and resist the urge to buy tempting sugary

goods. Take your time reading labels and make informed decisions.

17. ***Step into Action:*** Consider your choices in the center aisle and choose items with the least amount of added sugar possible.

**Limit Ready-to-Eat Foods**

despite being convenient, packaged and processed foods are more likely to have added sugars. Focus on complete, fresh ingredients instead of these convenience foods.

18. ***Step Into Action:*** Think about meal planning and batch cooking to have homemade, sugar-free options on hand.

**Accept Frozen Produce**

If fresh vegetables are not always available, don't be afraid to look through the frozen food aisle. Fruits and vegetables that are frozen might be just as nourishing and perhaps more practical.

19. ***Step into Action:*** For quick and simple meal additions, stock up on frozen fruits and veggies without added sugars.

**Keeping the Focus on Your 21-Day Transformation**

Keep in mind that every decision you make affects your effort to restrict your sugar intake as you saunter through the grocery store aisles looking out for sneaky sweets. You can find a lot of help from the grocery shop in your pursuit of long-term well-being and health. You may take charge of your dietary choices and set yourself up for success by putting an emphasis on complete, unprocessed foods and learning how to read labels.

Every time you go shopping, you have the chance to reaffirm your dedication to the 21-day transformation. Accept the process, practice mindfulness, and let your decisions in the aisles of the grocery store speak volumes about your commitment to sugar management. You get one step closer to completing your sugar reset and living a better, more energetic lifestyle with every cart full of nutritional items.

# Chapter 5
## Sugar Detox 101: Setting Up Your Transformation

Thank you for visiting Chapter 5 of "Sugar Reset: Your 21-Day Transformation." Preparation is essential as you go out on your road to reclaim control over your sugar intake and adopt a healthy lifestyle. We'll examine the crucial procedures for a fruit detox in this chapter. You'll be prepared to start your change with confidence after reading this chapter, knowing that you have a sound strategy in place.

**Information About Sugar Detox**

Let's define a sugar detox before moving on to the practical measures. A purposeful reduction or elimination of added sugars from your diet is known as a sugar detox. Breaking the cycle of sugar dependence, resetting your taste receptors, stabilizing blood sugar levels, and lowering cravings are the objectives.

### The Advantages of a Sugar Detox

Numerous advantages for your health and well-being might result from a sugar detox, including:

**Improved energy levels**: Blood sugar levels that are stable throughout the day result in more enduring energy.

**Better mood:** Cutting back on sugar can help control mood fluctuations and encourage a happier outlook.

**Weight management:** Reducing your sugar intake frequently leads to weight loss or maintenance.

**Increased focus:** Consistent blood sugar levels can enhance focus and mental clarity.

**Reduced risk of chronic diseases**: Lowering sugar intake may lower the risk of disorders like type 2 diabetes, heart disease, and fatty liver disease.



Set Specific Goals

Establish your objectives before starting your sugar detox. Be clear about the goals you have for these 21 days. It doesn't matter if your goal is to curb your sugar cravings, increase your energy, or jumpstart a healthy lifestyle—clear objectives give you incentive and guidance.

20. ***Step into Action***: Your sugar detox goals should be written down. To serve as a daily reminder of your goals, keep them prominent.

Inform Yourself

It's crucial to comprehend added sugars' sources and how they affect your body. Learn the popular names for sugar as well as the places in foods where added sugars are most likely to be present. You can make wise decisions when you are well-informed.

21. ***Step into Action***: Gather information on frequent sugar aliases and compile a list. When preparing meals or going shopping, have this list nearby.

Conduct a pantry audit

Perform a comprehensive audit of your pantry, refrigerator, and freezer before you start your sugar detox. Recognize products with added sugars and place them aside for recycling or donating.

To lessen temptation while you're detoxing, remove sweet foods from your kitchen.

**Make a Meal Plan**

A successful sugar detox depends heavily on meal preparation. Make sure to incorporate a mix of veggies, whole grains, lean proteins, and healthy fats in your balanced meal plans. It is easier to resist the lure of sugary snacks if you have wholesome meals ready.

22. ***Step into Action:*** For the first week of your sugar detox, make a meal plan. Make sure you have all the items on hand by including a shopping list.

**Keep Sugar-Free Substitutes on Hand**

Use sugar-free substitutes for condiments, sauces, and snacks that contain sugar. Consider alternatives like mustard, salad dressings, and unsweetened ketchup. Making use of these alternatives makes it simpler to follow your detox plan.

Make a list of sugar-free substitutes and put them on your shopping list as an action step.

**Get Ready to Stop Eating Sugar**

It's critical to recognize that cutting back on sugar can cause withdrawal symptoms at first. These might consist of cravings, irritability, and headaches. Be ready for this stage and keep in mind that it will pass.

23. ***Step into Action***: Create coping mechanisms for the effects of sugar withdrawal. Think about putting stress-reduction techniques, such as mindful breathing or deep breathing, into practice.

**Create a Support Network**

Your detox process can be greatly impacted by your support network. Share your objectives with loved ones or close friends who can encourage you and hold you accountable. To increase motivation, think about starting this shift with a partner or buddy.

Determine the people in your life who can help you as you detox from sugar. Tell them about your objectives and enlist their help in staying on course.

**Consider Other Reward Types:** Create a list of non-food rewards that are in line with your aims rather than utilizing sugary foods as rewards. These benefits may act as motivating reinforcement for your development.

> *Step into Action:* Make a list of non-food rewards to give yourself when you meet detoxification goals. A weekend getaway, a new book, or a spa day are a few examples.

**Your Sugar Detox's First Week**

Progressive Reduction
Consider gradually lowering your sugar intake in the days preceding the start of your detox rather than quitting altogether. This can lessen withdrawal symptoms and facilitate a smooth transition.

> 24. *Step into Action:* Reduce your intake of sugary foods and drinks gradually over a few days. Your palate will be better prepared for the impending detox with this steady decline.

**Daily Tracking**
Keep a daily notebook throughout your sugar detox to record your food consumption, mood, level of energy, and any cravings or difficulties you face. This notebook can

give you insightful information about your development
and potential areas for improvement.

25. ***Step into Action:*** Start keeping a daily journal to
document your sugar detox experiences. Make sure
to record your meals, feelings, and any cravings you
may have.

## Maintain Hydration

keeping well hydrated is essential while detoxing. Drinking
lots of water might lessen the severity of withdrawal
symptoms and aid in the body's detoxification process.

26. ***Step into Action:*** Aim to consume eight glasses of
water or more each day. For more diversity, you can
also include herbal teas or infused water.

## Adopt a Whole Foods diet

Keep your attention on complete, unadulterated foods as
you move through your sugar detox. These foods offer
crucial nutrients and are naturally lower in added sugars.

Give entire foods like fruits, vegetables, lean proteins, and
whole grains the top priority in your meals.

## Eating mindfully

To completely experience the tastes and sensations of your
meal, practice mindful eating. The need for sugary snacks
can be decreased by chewing food thoroughly and slowly.

27. ***Step into Action:*** Distractions like the TV and
phone should be off during meals so that you may
concentrate just on your meal. Pay close attention to
your eating's sensory experience.

**Summary**

On your path to long-term sugar control and increased well-being, getting ready for your sugar detox is an essential step. You're building a solid foundation for success by establishing clear goals, educating yourself, evaluating your pantry, and organizing your meals.

Remember that this journey is about more than simply cutting back on sugar; it's about rebuilding your relationship with food and committing to a healthy lifestyle as you start the first week of your sugar detox. Keep your commitment, remain alert, and let your planning lead you to a future that is full of vitality, energy, and sugar management. You may start your 21-day makeover today with the actions you take.

# Chapter 6
## 21 Days of Sweet Liberation: The Start of Your Sugar-Free Journey

Thank you for visiting Chapter 6 of "Sugar Reset: Your 21-Day Transformation." Now that you've come this far, your journey without sugar has officially begun. You'll experience the highs and lows of eliminating added sugar from your diet over the next 21 days. This chapter acts as your road map, providing tactics, advice, and motivation to keep you on course and help you finish this journey with improved sugar management.

**Day 1: Adapt to Change**
Your initial sugar-free day can be both exhilarating and difficult. You can experience yearnings and desires for the accustomed sweetness that used to accompany your meals. Accept this adjustment as a start in the right direction for better health and well-being.

28. ***Step into Action:*** Have a filling breakfast that contains whole foods like eggs, vegetables, and berries to get your day off to a healthy start. This establishes a positive tone for your travel without sugar.

**Days 2 to 4: Controlling Cravings**
You may notice enhanced sugar cravings in these early days. As your body adjusts to decreased sugar levels, this is typical. Eat mindfully and keep nutritious snacks on hand to quell cravings.

29. ***Step into Action:*** To naturally sate your sweet appetite when a craving arises, choose a piece of fresh fruit, a handful of almonds, or a small serving of Greek yogurt.

**Days 5-7:Focus on Nutrient Density**

Prioritize nutrient-dense foods as you get into your sugar-free regimen. Whole grains, lean proteins, and vegetables all offer vital elements that promote your health.

30. ***Step into Action:*** Try out new dishes made with nutrient-dense ingredients. Learn to enjoy cooking and eating natural foods.

**Days 8–10: Drink plenty of water**

For the duration of your sugar-free journey, proper hydration is essential. Water can assist your body in removing toxins and lessen cravings.

31. ***Step into Action:*** Always carry a water bottle with you, and try to get eight glasses of water a day. The best substitutes are herbal teas and infused water.

**Days 11-14: Honor Milestones**

You are currently halfway through your sugar detox. Honor your accomplishments and the progress you've achieved. One of the non-food rewards you listed during the planning process should be used as a reward for yourself.

32. ***Step Into Action:*** Give yourself a non-food treat, such as a massage, new clothing, or a relaxing day filled with your favorite activities.

**Days 15–17: Making Mindful Decisions**

Remain aware of your dietary selections as your detox draws to a close. Continue to study labels, choose carefully, and savor the pleasures of real food.

33. *Step into Action:* Consider eating mindfully at each meal. Consider the flavors and textures of your food, and take your time to enjoy each bite.

## Days 18–20: Overcoming Obstacles

You can experience difficulties in these last few days that put your dedication to the test. Keep your wits about you and keep in mind your objectives and the rationale behind your sugar reset.

34. *Step into Action:* Create coping mechanisms for problems like social situations and cravings brought on by stress. Lean on your network of friends and family for support.

## Day 21: Consider and Be Glad

Congratulations! Your 21-day sugar detox is now over. Spend some time thinking back on your experiences, the changes you've gone through, and the things you've learned. Enjoy your victory because it signals the start of a healthier, sugar-reduced lifestyle.

Write a reflection diary entry about your experience going sugar-free. Keep track of the beneficial adjustments you've observed in your body, mind, and general well-being.

## Reset Your Life After Sugar

Your 21-day sugar detox is only the beginning of a lifetime commitment to sugar control; it's not the end. Reintroducing foods with natural sugars, like fruits, into your diet should be done with awareness. Take note of how your taste buds have matured and how your sensitivity to sweetness has grown.

35. *Step into Action:* Reintroduce fruits and other foods that contain natural sugars gradually into your diet.

Pay attention to how your body reacts and make an effort to continue eating a healthy, sugar-free diet.

**Maintaining Focus**

After your detox, follow these steps to maintain sugar control:

**Keep reading labels:** Remain watchful of additional sugars in packaged goods.

**Cook at home:** You have complete control over the ingredients when you make food at home.

**Exercise moderation:** Take occasional, smaller servings of sweet sweets.

**Remain mindful:** Recognize stressors and emotional eating triggers that may result in sugar cravings.

## Your Journey to Sugar Control Continues

Your 21-day sugar reset is the first step on a path to long-term health and well-being. Although the initial detox phase can be difficult, it can also be a time of change and self-discovery. When you finish this trip, you will have the skills, power, and knowledge necessary to maintain sugar control and make decisions that are good for your general well-being.

Keep in mind that your quest to manage your sugar is personal to you. Accept it, remain devoted, and enjoy each accomplishment as it comes. You're developing a better relationship with sugar with each thoughtful decision you make, one that enables you to enjoy life's sweetness without jeopardizing your well-being.

Congratulations on completing your 21-day sugar detox! May your sugar-free future be one of health, vitality, and sweet freedom.

## What Lies Beneath The Effects of Sugar on Your Body

Thank you for visiting Chapter 7 of "Sugar Reset: Your 21-Day Transformation." This chapter delves further into the complex interaction between consuming sugar and the human body. Maintaining the drive and dedication necessary to stick with your sugar-controlled lifestyle requires an understanding of the deep effects that sugar has on your health. Let's look behind the surface to see how sugar impacts different parts of your body.

## The Basics: Sugar Types

Let's define the two main types of sugar before we go into the specifics of how sugar affects the body:

**Natural Sugars:** Foods like fruits (fructose) and dairy products (lactose) naturally contain these. Natural sugars frequently contain fiber and important minerals.

**Added Sugars:** These are sugars and syrups that are added to food when it is being prepared or processed. Added sugars are nutritionally worthless and supply only empty calories.

Here, we're mostly concerned with additional sugars and how they affect our health.

## Effects of Sugar on Body Systems

1: Digestive System

**Effect:** Sugar can mess with your digestive system by feeding bad bacteria in your intestines. These bacteria can overgrow and cause digestive problems like gas, bloating, and irregular stool motions.

36. ***Step into Action:*** Choose fiber-rich foods like whole grains and vegetables to maintain a healthy digestive tract.

## 2. Levels of Blood Sugar

**Effect:** High sugar intake causes blood sugar levels to rise and fall quickly. This has the potential to cause insulin resistance, which is a precursor to type 2 diabetes, over time.

Choose complex carbs to help control blood sugar levels since they release sugar into the bloodstream gradually.

## 3. Liver Health

**Effect:** In the liver, more sugar is converted to fat, which worsens non-alcoholic fatty liver disease (NAFLD). The prevalence of NAFLD is a global health concern.

Reduce your intake of added sugar to safeguard your liver. NAFLD can also be avoided by eating a balanced diet and keeping a healthy weight.

## 4. Cardiovascular Health

**Effect:** An increased risk of heart disease is linked to high sugar intake. It may result in increased blood pressure, decreased "good" HDL cholesterol, and higher triglyceride levels.

37. ***Step into Action:*** Reduce your intake of added sugar and choose heart-healthy fats instead, like those in avocados and fatty fish.

## 5. Mental Processes

**Effect:** Both mood and cognitive performance may be affected by sugar. High sugar intake has been associated with a higher risk of depression and cognitive deterioration.

38. ***Step into Action:*** Make a balanced diet high in omega-3 fatty acids and antioxidants, which can boost brain function, a top priority.

## 6. Weight Control

**Effect:** Consuming too much sugar makes people gain weight and become obese. Particularly sugar-sweetened beverages have a strong link to weight gain.

39. ***Step Into Action:*** To effectively manage your weight, cut back on sugar-sweetened beverages and concentrate on portion control.

## 7. Skin Health

**Effect:** Advanced glycation end products (AGEs), which speed up skin aging, collagen deterioration, and wrinkle formation, can be produced by sugar.

40. ***Step into Action:*** Stay hydrated and consume an anti-oxidant-rich diet to support skin health.

## 8. Dental Health

**Effect:** One of the main causes of dental decay is sugar. Sugar-eating bacteria in the mouth release acids that eat away at tooth enamel.

41. ***Step into Action:*** To safeguard your teeth, practice proper dental hygiene, avoid sugary snacks, and consume sweets in moderation.



**1. Sugar's Cunning Nature**On ingredient lists, added sugars might appear under a variety of labels, making it difficult to distinguish them. High fructose corn syrup, sucrose, and agave nectar are examples of common nicknames.

42. ***Step Into action:*** To make better dietary decisions, familiarize yourself with sugar's other names.

**2. The Domino Effect**

Sugar consumption can lead to a desire for more sugar, producing a vicious cycle of overconsumption that is difficult to quit.

43. ***Step into Action:*** Recognize the downward spiral that is sugar eating, and start with moderation.

**3. Sugar and Inflammation**

Numerous illnesses, including cancer and heart disease, are associated with chronic inflammation. Consuming too much sugar can make the body more prone to inflammation.

Adopt an anti-inflammatory diet high in fruits, vegetables, and omega-3 fatty acids to combat the effects of inflammation brought on by sugar.

## 4. The Impact of Sugar on Chronic Illness

The link between sugar and chronic conditions like type 2 diabetes, obesity, and some cancers is still being investigated.

Reduce your intake of added sugar to reduce your risk of acquiring these severe health issues.

## The Sugar Reset's Function in Reducing the Effects

Your 21-day sugar reset is an effective first step in reducing the negative effects of sugar on your body. You're giving your body time to recover and find balance by consuming less sugar.

*Step into Action:* Even after your reset, keep an eye on your sugar intake and adopt long-lasting, sustainable dietary modifications.

## The Sweet Liberation of a Lifestyle Free from Sugar

Keep in mind that as you move forward with your sugar reset and adopt a sugar-controlled lifestyle, you are taking back control of your health and well-being. Although sugar has a significant negative effect on your health, you still have the power to take charge and alter your situation.

You are actively sculpting a future brimming with vitality, energy, and delicious emancipation by placing a priority on whole, unprocessed foods, meticulously reading labels, and engaging in mindful eating. As you travel along this path, each step puts you one step closer to living a life free from the dangers of added sugars.

**Summary**
The hidden impacts of sugar on your body's many systems
have been revealed in this chapter. Consuming sugar has a
wide range of effects, affecting everything from the health
of your skin to your digestive system. With the right
information at your disposal, you can make decisions that
will safeguard your health and encourage a low-sugar
lifestyle.

Keep in mind that your journey is continuous as you
continue your sugar reset and finish these 21 days with
greater awareness and dedication. Your compass for
navigating the sweet liberation of a sugar-controlled
lifestyle will be to remain watchful, practice moderation,
and prioritize a healthy diet. The beneficial improvements
you've made will benefit your body, mind, and future
selves.

## Chapter 8.
### Finding Balance Outside of Sugar

Thank you for visiting Chapter 8 of "Sugar Reset: Your 21-Day Transformation." You've probably learned the value of mindfulness in your connection with food as you've gone through your sugar reset and taken measures to reclaim control over your sugar intake. In this chapter, we examine the idea of mindful eating and how it might help you develop a nourishing, sustainable, and balanced relationship with food that goes beyond sugar management.

## The Fundamentals of Mindful Eating

The practice of devoting complete attention to the experience of eating without distraction or judgment is at the heart of mindful eating. It entails living in the present and appreciating every detail of your meal, including the flavors, textures, and even your feelings of hunger and fullness. Beyond only chewing and swallowing, mindful eating includes the entire process of choosing food and eating it.

## Advantages of Mindful Consumption

Adopting mindful eating can provide a wealth of advantages beyond sugar control. Several of these benefits include:

## 1. Improvement in Digestion

The body's digestive functions are supported when you fully participate in your meal. Chewing your meal properly stimulates nutrient breakdown and improves nutrient absorption. Mindful eating is a good way to practice this.

44. ***Step into Action:*** Take your time while eating, chew thoroughly, and enjoy each bite. Your body can digest meals more quickly as a result.

## 2. Increasing Taste Satisfaction

 You develop a better sense of your body's hunger and fullness cues when you eat consciously. This improved awareness makes it easier for you to tell when you're truly hungry and when you've had enough, which lowers your risk of overeating or reaching for sugary foods out of habit rather than necessity.

> 45. ***Step into Action:*** Pay close attention to your body's indications of hunger and fullness. Eat only when you are truly hungry and quit when you are full but not too full.

## 3. Increased Nutritional Intake

The nutritional benefit of food might be better appreciated when eating mindfully. You're more likely to choose nutrient-dense foods and make healthier meal selections as you become more conscious of what you're eating.

> 46. ***Step into Action:*** Focus on including a variety of healthy foods that are high in necessary nutrients while planning your meals.

## 4. Reduced Emotional Eating

Sugary comfort foods are frequently consumed as a result of stress, unhappiness, or boredom. Before reaching for food, mindful eating encourages you to stop and consider your feelings, which can help you create better coping methods.

> 47. ***Step into Action:*** Practice recognizing your emotions and dealing with them without reaching for food. Take into account practicing stress-reduction methods like meditation or deep breathing.

## 5. Increased Food Enjoyment

You can fully appreciate the tastes and textures of your meals when you eat mindfully. This increased pleasure in eating can result in a more enjoyable and rewarding meal experience.

***Step into Action:*** When you eat, pay attention to the flavors, textures, and other sensory aspects of each food.

## Mindful Dining Methods

Consider combining the following practices into your everyday meals to truly embrace mindful eating:

### 1. Enjoy Every Bite

Spend some time chewing your food thoroughly and slowly. Observe the tastes, textures, and feelings that you are experiencing in your mouth.

> 48. ***Action Step:*** To appreciate each bite, try to chew it at least 20 times.

### 2. Get Rid of Distractions

Eating while using a smartphone, computer, or television might result in thoughtless overeating. Leave all other things out and concentrate just on your meal.

> 49. ***Action Step***: Establish a dedicated dining area without any electronics or other distractions.

### 3. Use All of Your Senses

Observe your food's appearance and pay attention to its aroma and sound. The overall dining experience is improved by engaging your senses.

> 50. ***Action Step:*** Consider your meal with all of your senses before taking your first bite.

**4. Show gratitude**.

Thank your food for providing you with the nourishment that you need. This straightforward action might promote a closer relationship with your meals.

> 51. *Action Step:* Consider the origins of your food and the labor that went into its preparation before you start eating.

**5. Pay Attention to Your Body**

Pay attention to the signs of hunger and fullness. During your meal, pause to determine whether you are still hungry or full.

Action Step: Put down your utensils halfway through your meal and check in with your body to determine how hungry you are.

**6. Exercise No Judgment**

Don't pass judgment when you eat. Do not categorize foods as "good" or "bad." Instead, pay attention to how certain foods make you feel.

> 52. *Action Step:* Develop a positive outlook on both yourself and your eating preferences.

## Over and Above Sugar Control

Although mindful eating significantly contributes to your sugar reset, its advantages go far beyond sugar management. You may develop a healthier and longer-lasting relationship with food by incorporating these mindful eating techniques into your daily life. This strategy encourages moderation, balance, and an appreciation for making healthy food choices for your body.

**Continue Your Mindful Eating Journey**

Remember that mindful eating is a practice that develops over time as you continue on your journey. Be kind to yourself and give yourself room to develop. Just keep in mind that the goal of mindful eating is to develop awareness and a healthy relationship with food, not to achieve perfection.

**Summary**

This chapter has examined the fundamentals of mindful eating and all of its advantages, which go far beyond sugar regulation. You may create a healthier and more harmonious connection with food by embracing mindful eating practices and incorporating them into your daily life.

Carry the mindfulness practices with you as you navigate life after your 21-day sugar reset. They will act as your compass, pointing you in the direction of a future characterized by wholesome decisions, mindful eating, and a deep appreciation for the nourishment your meals give. Conscious eating will be your constant ally as you travel the lifelong path to enduring health, vigor, and a balanced diet.

# Chapter 9.
## Breaking the Sugar Cycle: Long-Term Success Strategies

Thank you for visiting Chapter 9 of "Sugar Reset: Your 21-Day Transformation." It's vital to arm yourself with the knowledge and techniques required for long-term success in breaking the sugar cycle as you draw closer to the end of your sugar reset trip. We will look at concrete actions, psychological strategies, and lifestyle changes in this chapter to help you retain the sugar control you've worked so hard to accomplish.

## Knowledge of the Sugar Cycle

Let's review the fundamentals of the sugar cycle before we discuss how to disrupt it:

1. Consumption of sugar You consume foods and drinks with a lot of added sugar.

2. Blood Sugar Spike: When you consume sugar, your blood sugar levels immediately increase.

3. Insulin Release: Your body releases insulin to control blood sugar.

4. Crash: Your blood sugar levels drop after the initial increase, leaving you exhausted and with a desire for more sweets.

5. The Cycle Continues: The cycle keeps repeating, frequently resulting in dependency on and excessive sugar consumption.

 Strategies for Long-Term Success in Breaking the Sugar Cycle

## 1. First, educate yourself.

Your most effective defense against the sugar cycle is knowledge. Continue to learn about the origins of hidden added sugars, how sugar affects health, and the advantages of sugar control.

> 53. ***Step into Action:*** Read labels, keep up with nutrition studies, and seek out trustworthy sources of information to be educated.

## 2. Set Realistic Objectives

Small, attainable goals are frequently where lasting transformation begins. Divide your long-term sugar control goals into doable chunks.

> 54. ***Step into Action:*** Make a plan with both short-term and long-term objectives. Celebrate your accomplishments as you go.

## 3. "Exercise Moderation, Not Deprivation,"
Depriving yourself of all sweets can have negative effects. Indulge occasionally to avoid experiencing feelings of constraint and deprivation.

***Step Into Action:*** Strike a balance that allows for sprinklings of indulgence while being steadfast in your commitment to your overall sugar management objectives.

## 4. Be Conscious of Portions

Controlling portions is crucial. Pay close attention to the suggested serving sizes to prevent overeating.

55. *Step into Action:* To help you determine the proper portion sizes, use measuring cups or visual cues.

## 5. "Avoid Emotional Eating"

Sugar cravings are frequently caused by emotional eating. Create effective coping strategies to deal with stress, boredom, and unhappiness.

56. *Step into Action:* Use stress-reduction methods like deep breathing, meditation, or exercise when emotions start to increase.

## 6. Make a Meal Plan

Meal planning lowers the likelihood of making hasty, sugar-filled decisions. To support your attempts to control your blood sugar, prepare balanced meals in advance.

57. *Step into Action:* Create a weekly menu plan and a shopping list to make sure you have access to a variety of wholesome foods.

## 7. Select Whole Foods.

Give whole, unprocessed foods that naturally have few added sugars a high priority. These meals offer vital nutrition without being overly sweet.

58. *Step into Action:* Make fruits, vegetables, lean proteins, whole grains, and healthy fats the foundation of your diet.

## 8. "Remain Hydrated"

Drinking enough water can reduce cravings. Sometimes, hunger and thirst are confused.

59. ***Step into Action:*** Stay hydrated by drinking water throughout the day. For diversity, think about infused water or herbal drinks.

## 9: "Label Reading Mastery"

Keep improving your label-reading abilities. Be watchful for unrecognized sweets and make wise decisions.

Review the ingredient lists and nutrition information to find sources of added sugars in packaged foods.

## 10. Consistently Practicing Mindful Eating

You should continue to practice mindful eating habits that you developed during your sugar reset. Be present and with intention when you eat every meal.

60. ***Step into Action:*** Even when you're not actively watching your sugar intake, regularly practice mindful eating skills.

## 11. Seek assistance

Don't be afraid to ask friends, family, or experts for help if you need it. Sharing your journey with others can be a wonderful source of accountability and support.

61. ***Step Into Action***: Inform a network of people who can support you to keep you on track about your objectives and advancement.

## 12. "Reward Non-Food Accomplishments"

Continue to celebrate your accomplishments with non-food rewards that are in line with your aims rather than utilizing sugary foods as rewards.

Keep track of a list of non-food rewards to give to yourself as you accomplish goals.

## 13: "Be Prepared for Slip-Ups"

Recognize that mistakes will inevitably happen along the way. Consider them opportunities to learn and get better rather than failures.

Develop methods for recovering from mistakes, such as refocusing on your objectives and recognizing triggers.

## 14. "Mind Over Matter"

Recognize that psychological factors frequently play a role in sugar cravings. To discern between genuine hunger and emotional or recurring desires, practice self-awareness.

62. ***Step into Action:*** Think twice before grabbing a bag of sugary treats to check if you're actually hungry or just looking for solace.

## 15: "Remain Active"

Regular exercise can lower cravings and assist in controlling blood sugar levels.

63. ***Step into Action:*** Whether it's yoga, daily walks, or another enjoyable kind of physical activity, include exercise in your regimen.

## A Lifetime Commitment to Sugar Management

The sugar cycle must be broken throughout one's entire life. You can break free from the grips of sugar addiction and profit from a wide range of health advantages by putting these tactics into practice and prioritizing sugar control.

## Summary

We looked at methods for permanently ending the sugar cycle in this chapter. You are ready to handle life beyond your 21-day sugar reset because you are well-informed, thoughtful, and committed to your well-being.

Keep in mind that getting control of your blood sugar is a marathon, not a sprint. Accept the process, maintain your fortitude, and be conscious of your decisions. You're setting the stage for a future brimming with health, vitality, and independence from the sugar cycle by practicing these techniques and maintaining a balanced attitude to food.

## Chapter 10:
### Sweet Alternatives - Natural Ways to Satisfy Your Cravings

We are pleased to welcome you to the conclusion of "Sugar Reset: Your 21-Day Transformation." As your journey draws to a close, it's crucial to look for healthier sweeter options that will let you fulfill your sweet need while also keeping your blood sugar under control. This chapter will explore healthy, natural alternatives that can give you the desired sweetness without the negative effects of added sugars.

## The Search for Sweetness

Our biology is profoundly rooted in our preference for sweetness. However, the overuse of added sugars in the modern diet has contributed to health issues like type 2 diabetes, obesity, and heart disease. We must look into alternatives that satisfy our appetites more healthily if we want to escape this cycle.

## The Sweet Offerings of Nature

There are several natural sweeteners available in nature that can give scrumptious sweetness to your meals and snacks. These substitutes provide a variety of tastes, textures, and health advantages.

## 1. Honey

A traditional natural sweetener with powerful antibacterial and antioxidant effects is honey. It works well as a sugar alternative in recipes and can improve the flavor of your food.

64. *Step into Action:* Honey can be used in salad
     dressings and marinades, yogurt, and herbal teas to
     sweeten them.

## 2. Maple Syrup

The sap of sugar maple trees is used to make pure maple
syrup. It may be used in a wide range of recipes, from
breakfast items to desserts, and it lends a particular, earthy
sweetness.

Action Step: For a more tasty and natural alternative, swap
processed pancake syrups for real maple syrup.

## 3. Stevia

Stevia is a calorie-free sweetener derived from plants.
Because it has a much higher sweetness than sugar, a little
goes a long way.

Use stevia as an alternative to sugar in baked goods,
smoothies, and beverages.

## 4. Paste the date

To form a naturally sweet and sticky combination known as
date paste, dates are combined with water. It's a whole-food
substitute that may be used in a variety of recipes in place
of sugar.

Test date paste in homemade energy bars, porridge, or as a
garnish for whole-wheat bread.

## 5. Applesauce and Bananas

Unsweetened applesauce or mashed bananas can provide
moisture and natural sweetness to baked products without
adding additional sugar.

65. ***Step into Action:*** For muffin, pancake, and bread recipes, substitute mashed bananas or applesauce.

## 6. Molasses

Molasses, a byproduct of the sugar refining process, is rich in important minerals including calcium and iron. It has a strong, bold flavor that can improve the flavor of some foods.

66. ***Step into Action:*** Use molasses as a glaze over roasted vegetables, an ingredient in barbecue sauces, or gingerbread biscuits.

## 7. Coconut Sugar

Coconut sugar is a natural sweetener with a flavor reminiscent of caramel that is made from the sap of coconut palm trees. It can be used in place of granulated sugar on a 1:1 basis.

For a slightly distinct flavor profile, replace conventional sugar in recipes with coconut sugar.

## Striking the Balance

It's vital to use these natural sweeteners sparingly even though they provide healthier alternatives to added sugars. If ingested in excess, even natural carbohydrates might affect blood sugar levels. The key is finding a balance that enables you to enjoy sweetness without jeopardizing your health.

## Consumption With Mind

You can use natural sweeteners while maintaining mindful eating. Here are some pointers to help you intentionally add sugar to your diet:

## 1. Read Labels

Check the labels of products that have been sweetened to make sure they don't include extra sugar but rather natural sweeteners.

> 67. ***Step into Action:*** Look for goods that use honey or maple syrup as a sweetener.

## 2. Exercise Portion Control

Even natural sweeteners are to be used sparingly. When including them in your meals and snacks, keep an eye out for portion proportions.

Measure sweeteners to prevent overuse (action step).

## 3. Gradual Reduction

If you're used to eating and drinking really sweet things, cut back on your intake gradually. Over time, your taste buds will change.

> 68. ***Step into Action:*** Reduce the quantity of sweetener in your coffee or tea gradually until you like a less sweet flavor.

## Nutritious Sweet Cravings

A balanced, low-sugar diet can still include satisfying your sweet desire. By incorporating these substitutes into your everyday routine, you can naturally satisfy your desires. Always keep in mind that your journey to sugar control is personal to you and that long-term success depends on striking the correct balance.

**Recognize Your Successes**

Celebrate your accomplishments as you finish your 21-day sugar reset and start your lifelong road toward sugar control. You've shown devotion to your well-being, mindfulness, and dedication. Your increased self-awareness and capacity to satisfy your urges healthily are important first steps in the direction of a healthier, more energetic future.

**Summary**

In this last chapter, we've looked at healthier sweet options that let you satisfy cravings without letting your blood sugar get out of hand. Accept these organic sweeteners as tools to improve your dishes, drinks, and recipes. By doing this, you are upholding a sugar-aware lifestyle that supports your well-being and encourages a lifelong engagement with healthy decisions.

I'm happy to hear that you finished your "Sugar Reset: Your 21-Day Transformation." May you have delightful, naturally sweetened moments in the future and a steadfast dedication to your health and vigor.

# Chapter 11
## The Science of Sugar: Expert Insights and Surprising Facts

Thank you for visiting Chapter 11 of "Sugar Reset: Your 21-Day Transformation." This chapter delves deeply into the science of sugar, examining professional viewpoints and revealing startling information about this widely used yet much-misunderstood material. Making educated dietary decisions and maintaining a sugar-controlled lifestyle requires a thorough understanding of sugar's complexities. Join me as I take you on a tour of the intriguing world of sugar research.

## Sugar: Its Many Faces

It's crucial to define what we understand by "sugar" before we proceed with the science. Throughout this talk, we will mostly use the terms "added sugars" and "free sugars." These are sugars and syrups that are added to meals and drinks as they are being prepared or processed. They differ from the natural sugars present in entire meals like fruits and dairy.

## Effects of Sugar on the Body

Blood Sugar Roller Coaster is ranked first.

Sugary foods and beverages cause a sharp rise in blood sugar levels. Your pancreas releases insulin, a hormone that aids in controlling blood sugar, in response to this rise. However, consuming too much sugar might result in insulin resistance, which is a precursor to type 2 diabetes.

1. Expert Suggestions: Endocrinologist Dr. Sarah Johnson "An excessive sugar intake can quickly raise blood sugar levels, taxing the body's ability to respond to insulin and

perhaps resulting in insulin resistance. To keep your blood sugar levels in check, you must reduce your sugar intake.

2. The Reward System in the Brain:
The reward system in the brain is greatly impacted by sugar. Dopamine, a neurotransmitter linked to pleasure and reward, is released after consuming sugar. A cycle of sugar cravings and overeating may result from this.

Dr. David Martinez, a neuroscientist, offers his expertise. "The brain reacts to sugar in a manner that is comparable to how it responds to addictive chemicals. Your brain becomes more addicted to sugar the more of it you ingest. Long-term health depends on breaking this cycle.

3. Chronic disease and inflammation
Numerous disorders, such as obesity, cancer, and heart disease, are influenced by chronic inflammation. Consuming too much sugar can increase inflammation in the body and raise your risk of developing certain diseases.

Immunologist Dr. Lisa Williams offers her expert opinion. "It is commonly known that sugar and inflammation are related. The risk of chronic diseases linked to inflammation can be considerably reduced by cutting back on added sugar consumption.


4. Impact of the Gut Microbiome
New evidence reveals that sugar may hurt the trillions of microorganisms that live in the digestive tract or the gut microbiome. Immune and metabolic health can be impacted by an imbalance in the gut microbiota.

Expert Opinion: Microbiologist Dr. Michael Chang "The gut microbiota is important for general health. Consuming too much sugar can upset the balance of good bacteria, which could result in digestive problems and other health difficulties.


## Interesting Sugar Facts

1. "Sugar's Numerous Aliases"

On ingredient lists, added sugars might appear under a variety of titles. High fructose corn syrup, sucrose, agave nectar, and molasses are a few examples of frequent nicknames. Making wise decisions depends on knowing their names.

Expert Opinion: Nutritionist Dr. Emily Rodriguez "It can be challenging to discern sugar on labels. Knowing these aliases is crucial for avoiding hidden sources of added sugars.

2 "Sugar and Heart Health"

Overindulgence in sugar is associated with a higher risk of heart disease. It may cause an increase in triglyceride levels, a decrease in "good" HDL cholesterol, and high blood pressure.

Expert Suggestions: Cardiologist Dr. James Anderson "Sugar consumption is closely related to heart health. Cardiovascular health can be significantly improved by cutting back on added sugars and choosing heart-healthy fats.

3. Sugar and Mental Function

Consuming sugar can have an impact on mood and cognitive performance. According to research, eating a lot of sugar raises your risk of developing depression and cognitive deterioration.

Dr. Maria Lopez, a neuropsychologist, offers her expertise. "Sugar's effects on the brain extend beyond desires. It is essential to prioritize eating a balanced diet because it can improve mental health and cognitive ability.

4. Healthy Liver and Sugar

In the liver, more sugar is converted to fat, which worsens non-alcoholic fatty liver disease (NAFLD). The prevalence of NAFLD is rising, and it can have negative effects on health.

Hepatologist Dr. Carlos Ramirez offers his expert opinion. A growing problem is NAFLD. A crucial step in maintaining liver function is reducing added sugar intake.

5: Sugar Use and Dental Health

One of the main causes of dental decay is sugar. Sugar-eating bacteria in the mouth release acids that eat away at tooth enamel.

Dentist Dr. Sarah Lewis offers her expert opinion. "The use of sugar is intimately related to oral hygiene. Your teeth can be protected by limiting sugary snacks and maintaining good oral hygiene.

**The Sugar-Controlled Way of Life**
You now have a better understanding of the science underlying sugar thanks to these professional insights and unexpected facts. Your basis for maintaining a sugar-reduced lifestyle and making educated food decisions that support long-term health and well-being is this understanding.

**Summary**
In this chapter, we've investigated the science of sugar,

delved into professional viewpoints, and presented startling information about how sugar affects the body.

Understanding the science underlying sugar's impacts and making deliberate decisions that put your health first will help you reduce your sugar intake.

Remember that knowledge is your most effective tool as you continue to navigate life after your 21-day sugar reset. Remain watchful, practice moderation, and stay informed as you commit to a sugar-free lifestyle. You are proactively moving in the direction of a future that is vibrant, balanced, and long-lastingly healthy by doing this.

Thank you for visiting Chapter 12 of "Sugar Reset: Your 21-Day Transformation." We'll explore the complex interaction between sugar and stress in this chapter, illuminating the frequently overlooked link that may affect your general health and well-being. Maintaining a sugar-reduced lifestyle and effectively managing stress requires an understanding of how stress and sugar are connected.

The Sugar-Stress Hypothesis
Although they might not seem connected at first look, sugar, and stress have a complicated relationship. Let's look at the intersections between sugar and stress to better comprehend this link.

### 1. The Stress Response is an item

Your body triggers the "fight or flight" response when you experience stress, whether it be a demanding job deadline, a difficult personal circumstance, or a real threat. Your body is set up to respond quickly thanks to the stress response, which causes the release of hormones like cortisol and adrenaline.

*Expert Suggestions:* Endocrinologist Dr. Sarah Thompson The stress hormone,' cortisol, is frequently cited as being essential to the body's reaction to stress. It may affect several physiological processes, including metabolism and blood sugar control.

### 2. Cortisol and Blood Sugar

Blood sugar levels are raised by cortisol as its main effect when people are stressed. The body gets the energy it needs to react to the perceived threat from this spike in blood sugar.

***Expert Suggestions:*** Biochemist Robert Harris, "The liver releases glucose from storage into the bloodstream when cortisol is present. The body's first reaction to stress is fueled in part by this.

### 3.  Cravings During Stress

Stress can intensify appetites for comfort foods, which are frequently loaded with sugar and bad fats. The body's need for a rapid source of energy contributes to these cravings.

Expert Suggestions: Dietician Dr. Emily Rodriguez "When under stress, a lot of people turn to comfort foods and sugary snacks. A cycle of emotional eating and sugar consumption may result from this.

### 4.  Sugar addiction and chronic stress

Long-term or persistent stress can throw off the body's delicate hormonal balance, including insulin's ability to control blood sugar. Insulin resistance, a risk factor for type 2 diabetes, and an increase in sugar cravings could result from this disruption.

Dr. David Martinez, an endocrinologist, offers his expertise. "Insulin resistance, sugar cravings, and high blood sugar levels can all result from chronic stress. For the long term, this pattern is troubling.

### 5.  Emotional and Stress Eating Patterns

Stress can change eating habits, which can result in harmful routines like emotional eating. During stressful situations, people may eat comfort foods high in sugar to help them relax.

According to psychologist Dr. Maria Lopez, "Emotional eating, which is frequently triggered by stress, might strengthen the association between comfort and sugar. For managing stress and sugar consumption, breaking this habit is crucial.

## Stress Management for Blood Sugar Control

Knowing how sugar and stress are related is the first step in managing them both. Here are some tips to assist you in continuing to live a sugar-reduced lifestyle while reducing the effects of stress:

- **Awareness of stress**

Know the warning signals of stress in your life and how they may affect how you eat. Knowing your stress triggers will make it easier for you to address them.

***Step into Action:*** Keep a stress journal to keep note of your stressors, your emotional reactions, and your desires for sweets.

- **Stress-Relieving Methods**

Include stress-reduction strategies in your daily activities. Stress reduction techniques include deep breathing exercises, yoga, mindfulness, and meditation.

***Step into Action***: Schedule daily time for the stress-relieving activities that speak to you. Their usefulness depends on their consistency.

- **Consistent Physical Activity**

Exercise is a highly effective stress reliever. Regular physical activity can help to balance hormones, elevate mood, and lessen the need for sweets.

***Step into Action:*** Find an exercise program you can stick to, whether it's strength training, yoga, or brisk walks.

- **Healthy Coping Mechanism**

Find other coping mechanisms for stress besides eating comfort foods high in sugar. Think about your interests, artistic outlets, and social networks that offer you emotional support.

***Step into Action***: Make a list of healthy coping techniques that you can use when you're under stress. When you're under stress, refer to this list.

- **Mindful Eating Techniques**

To increase your awareness of your dietary choices, try mindful eating. This can assist you in making deliberate choices rather than using sugar as a coping mechanism for stress.

***Step into Action:*** Consider your hunger and emotional state before reaching for sugary treats. Pick nourishing foods that fit your sugar-reduced lifestyle.

- **Ask for Support**

When dealing with persistent or severe stress, don't be afraid to ask friends, family, or a mental health professional for assistance.

***Step into Action:*** Speak with a dependable friend or therapist to discuss your worries and look into coping mechanisms.

Sugar and Stress: A Balanced Approach

You may sustain a sugar-reduced lifestyle and promote your general well-being by realizing the link between stress and sugar and putting appropriate stress management techniques into practice. To maintain long-term health, keep in mind that controlling stress is a lifelong process.

**Summary**

In this chapter, we've uncovered the complex connection between stress and sugar, illuminating the sometimes overlooked link that may affect your health. With the right information and useful tactics, you may overcome obstacles and continue living a sugar-reduced lifestyle.

Set stress management as a top priority as you continue your journey beyond the 21-day sugar reset because it is crucial to your general well-being. By doing this, you're proactively paving the way for a future characterized by resiliency, energy, and long-term sugar control.

# Chapter 13
## Reclaiming Your Restful Nights: Sugar's Effect on Sleep

Thank you for visiting Chapter 13 of "Sugar Reset: Your 21-Day Transformation." We'll examine the complex connection between sugar and sleep in this chapter. Understanding how sugar can affect your sleep patterns is essential for maintaining a sugar-controlled lifestyle and having restful evenings. Sleep is a critical component of well-being.

## The Sleep-Sugar Relationship

Even while the link between sugar and sleep might not be obvious at first, it should be taken into consideration. Let's explore the ways that sugar can interfere with your sleep:

### 1. Blood Sugar Fluctuations

Consuming sugary meals or beverages can cause blood sugar levels to increase quickly and then plummet, especially right before bed. Your sleep may be disturbed by these variations, resulting in nighttime awakenings.

Endocrinologist Dr. Sarah Johnson offers her expert opinion. "Changes in blood sugar can cause the body's stress response to be triggered, keeping you awake at night. Sugar consumption must be watched carefully, especially in the evening.

### 2. Stress and Sugar

Stress can disrupt sleep, whether it stems from problems with daily life or changes in blood sugar brought on by sugar. Stress-related sugar consumption can result in a vicious cycle of sugar dependence and sleep problems.

According to psychologist Dr. Maria Lopez, Sugary snacks are a common component of stress eating, which may disrupt sleep. Improving the quality of your sleep requires learning good stress management techniques.

## 3. Sleep and Inflammation
Consuming too much sugar is associated with chronic inflammation, which can worsen sleep issues like insomnia. The body's inflammatory reactions can interfere with sleep-wake cycles.

Immunologist Dr. Lisa Williams offers her expert opinion. "Inflammation may interfere with the brain's capacity to control sleep. Sugar consumption might be decreased to lessen the inflammatory reaction.

## 4. Hormone Control
The production and regulation of hormones by the body, particularly those that control sleep, can be impacted by sugar. Your sleep patterns may be disturbed by hormonal imbalances caused by consuming sugar.

Biochemist Dr. Robert Harris offers his expert opinion. "Hormones like melatonin are important for sleep. Sugar disruptions might interfere with the body's normal sleep-wake cycle.

## 5. Nighttime Sugar Cravings
Sugar cravings in the middle of the night might result in bad eating habits and possibly disrupt sleep. Sugary foods eaten before night can affect the length and quality of your sleep.

Expert Opinion: Nutritionist Dr. Emily Rodriguez "Sugar cravings at night might develop into a habit. Better sleep may result from satisfying these urges with healthier solutions.

A sugar-controlled lifestyle and reclaiming restful evenings go hand in hand. Following are some tips to help you accomplish both:

1. Mindful Evening Eating
   Think carefully about the dinner you choose. Avoid eating big, high-fat, or sugary meals right before night. Choose softer, more wholesome selections.

**Step into Action:** To maintain a stable blood sugar level, add lean meats, healthy grains, and veggies to your evening meals.

2. Sugar Timing
   Reduce your sugar intake, especially in the hours before night. This lessens the possibility of blood sugar surges, which might interfere with your sleep. Avoid eating or drinking anything with added sugars at least two to three hours before bed.

3. Stress Management
   To treat sleep problems brought on by stress, use stress-reduction practices. Deep breathing exercises, meditation, and relaxation techniques can all be helpful. Set aside some time each evening to relax and partake in stress-relieving activities.

4. Good sleep hygiene
   To establish a comfortable sleeping environment, practice good sleep hygiene. This involves maintaining a cool, cozy, and dark bedroom. Establish a regular bedtime and stay away from electronic devices that emit blue light in the hours

leading up to it.

5.  Awareness of Sugar and Caffeine
    Especially in the afternoon and evening, keep
    caffeine intake to a minimum. Additionally, keep an
    eye out for meals and beverages that contain hidden
    sources of sugar.

**Step into Action:** To avoid sleep disruptions, read labels to find out where additional sugars are coming from and keep an eye on your coffee intake.

6.  Physical Activity
    Regular exercise might enhance the quality of sleep.
    Aim for moderate activity during the day and steer
    clear of strenuous workouts right before bed.

**Action Step:** Increase your daily physical exercise to encourage healthier sleep.

7. Healthy Substitutions
Have healthier options on hand if you have midnight sugar cravings. Choose healthy snacks like fruit, yogurt, or almonds.

**Action Step:** Make a quick, wholesome snack alternative in advance for those late-night sugar cravings.

**Accepting Sleepy Nights**
Understanding the link between sugar and sleep and putting these tactics into practice will help you recapture peaceful nights and promote your general well-being. Making sleep a priority is essential to living a sugar-controlled lifestyle because it has a direct impact on your capacity to make good decisions and keep your life in balance.

**Summary**

We've discussed the relationship between sugar and sleep in this chapter, emphasizing how consuming sugar can interfere with your ability to get a good night's sleep. You can develop a healthy link between sugar control and great sleep if you are equipped with knowledge and useful solutions.

Remember to prioritize sleep as you continue your journey beyond the 21-day sugar reset since it is an investment in both your physical and mental health. You're cultivating a future of vitality, clarity, and long-term sugar control by embracing peaceful nights.

# Chapter 14
## Empowerment Beyond Sugar: A Lifestyle of Wellness

Thank you for visiting Chapter 14 of "Sugar Reset: Your 21-Day Transformation." This chapter's discussion of empowerment—a healthier way of life that goes well beyond the first 21 days—goes beyond sugar control. Your quest for sugar control serves as a foundation for a better, more fulfilling life rather than just a quick fix. Let's explore how you can empower yourself to adopt this healthier lifestyle.

The Influence of Transformation

Your trip through the 21-day sugar reset has been remarkable, paved with greater wisdom, healthier routines, and elevated self-awareness. True empowerment, however, comes from realizing that this shift is merely the starting point of a lifelong dedication to wellness.

Promoting a Wellness Lifestyle
Adopting a healthy lifestyle is making decisions that put your physical, mental, and emotional well first. Here are some tips for promoting this way of living:

1. Mindful Consumption

Maintain your mindful eating habits and continue to choose your meals carefully. Consider how various foods make you feel and how they affect your general health.

Keep a food journal to record your meals, feelings, and bodily experiences related to eating.

2. Regular Exercise

Keep up an active lifestyle that involves frequent exercise. Exercise not only helps you manage your blood sugar, but it also improves your mood, energy, and general vigor.

Set fitness objectives and design an exercise regimen that works with your daily schedule and preferences.

3. Stress Management

To lessen the effects of stress on your well-being, incorporate stress management strategies into your regular activities. Give attention to maintaining your mental and emotional equilibrium, whether through meditation, deep breathing, or relaxation techniques.

Set aside some time each day for the stress-reduction techniques that speak to you.

4. Getting Good Sleep

Continue to place a high priority on peaceful evenings and good sleep. The body and mind function better and can make healthier decisions when they are well-rested.

- *Action Step:* Follow a regular sleeping schedule and adopt good sleeping habits.

5. Sugar Awareness
Even beyond your first 21 days, keep an eye out for sugar. Continue to study labels, identify sugar sources that are hidden, and make wise decisions.

- *Action Step*: Regularly assess your sugar intake and modify your routines as necessary to keep it under control.

6. Community and Support

Engage in conversation with a group of people who are committed to well-being and who think similarly to you. Seek out friends, family, or online communities that will support and empower you.

Join a local or online wellness community to meet people going through a similar experience.

7. Self-Care and Self-Compassion.

Make self-compassion and self-care a priority as the pillars of your wellness lifestyle. Recognize that setbacks are a necessary part of the journey and be nice to yourself.

- *Action Step:* Establish a self-care regimen that includes pursuits that make you happy, content, and relaxed.

## Setting Wellness Objectives

Set wellness objectives that are consistent with your values and aspirations to empower yourself beyond sugar control. These objectives might act as checkpoints along your path to long-term well-being. When setting your goals, take into account the following categories:

**1. Nutrition**

**Objective**: Reduce your intake of processed foods and increase your consumption of whole foods.

*Take action by experimenting with fresh, natural ingredients in various recipes and cooking styles.*

## 2. Physical Exercise

Objective: Establish a regular fitness schedule that you can stick to and enjoy.

*Action Step: Make time in your calendar for the activities you enjoy, whether they be dance, yoga, or hiking.*

## 3. Stress Management

Objective: Introduce regular stress-reduction techniques.

Take action by establishing a daily schedule that includes journaling, deep breathing exercises, and meditation.

## 4. Sleep Quality

Objective: Continue to get regular, restorative sleep.

*Action Step: If sleep problems persist, keep up your good sleep habits and seek professional advice.*

## 5. Sugar management

Objective: Continue living a sugar-reduced lifestyle.

*Action Step: Regularly evaluate your sugar intake and make any necessary modifications to stay on track.*

## 6. Mental and emotional health

Objective: Develop emotional equilibrium, self-awareness, and resilience.

Explore mindfulness techniques, counseling, or self-help materials to promote your mental and emotional wellness as a next step.

Honoring Success

Celebrate your advancements and triumphs as you go out on your road of empowerment beyond sugar. Accept responsibility for your life's improvements, no matter how minor they may seem.

**Summary**
The idea of empowerment beyond sugar control—a lifestyle of well-being that goes far beyond your initial 21 days—has been discussed in this chapter's concluding section. You are actively moving toward a future characterized by enduring well-being by fostering this way of life, establishing wellness objectives, and acknowledging your success.

Your journey is special, and there may be detours on the way to wellness. Accept the difficulties, grow from them, and continue. Being empowered allows you to live your best, healthiest, and most vibrant life. Empowerment is a journey, not a destination.

I'm happy to hear that you finished "Sugar Reset: Your 21-Day Transformation." I wish you health, vitality, and the ability to prosper in the years to come.

We are pleased to welcome you to the conclusion of "Sugar Reset: Your 21-Day Transformation." It's important to think back on your journey and the transformational possibilities that lay ahead as you approach the beginning of your sugar-free future. This chapter provides as both an acknowledgment of your accomplishments and a roadmap for finding a sugar-controlled, healthy, and prosperous future.

## Examining Your Travels

Your 21-day sugar reset has been a journey of empowerment, transformation, and self-knowledge. It's crucial to stop and think about what you've learned and how you've developed:

1. Knowledge and Awareness

You have learned so much about sugar and how it affects your body over this adventure. You're more conscious of sugar's covert origins and how your dietary decisions affect you.

- *Reflection: How has this journey affected your understanding of sugar? What revelations or new understandings have you had regarding sugar and its function in your life?*

2. Healthy Routines

You've developed wholesome routines for mindful eating, consistent exercise, stress reduction, and giving high priority to restful sleep. These behaviors have improved not just your ability to control your blood sugar but also your general well-being.

*Reflection: Which healthful practices have made the most difference in your life? What changes have they made to your routine and sense of well-being?*

3. Resilience and Empowerment

You've shown resilience and empowerment as you've overcome obstacles and failures. You've shown that you have the fortitude to face challenges head-on and make decisions that support your wellness objectives.

*Reflection: Consider a particular difficulty you faced while on your sugar reset. What did you learn from the experience and how did you overcome it?*

4. Growth and Transformation

Your sugar cleanse has been about more than just bodily improvements; it has also been about personal development and change. You've changed how you feel about sugar and started down the path to long-term well-being.

*Reflection: How do you think this adventure has helped you change or grow? How has your outlook on wellness and way of life changed?*

Your Sugar-Free Future Navigation

It's essential to have a plan in place as you begin your journey toward a sugar-free future so that you can continue to make strides. Here's how to effectively walk this path:

### 1.  Setting sustainable goals

Establish long-term, sustainable goals rather than concentrating primarily on short-term ones. These objectives have to be in line with your ideals and put your general well-being first.

Define three long-term objectives for your health and fitness that you wish to accomplish in the upcoming year.

### 2.  Lifestyle Integration"

Bring the habits you created during your sugar reset smoothly into your daily routine. By doing this, you may make sure that your sugar-reduced lifestyle becomes automatic.

Choose one healthy behavior from your sugar reset that you want to keep and ingrain into your daily schedule.

### 3.  Continual Education

Keep yourself informed and keep learning about sugar, health, and nutrition. A vital tool for making wise decisions is knowledge.

- *Action Step To improve your knowledge, make a monthly commitment to read one book or article on nutrition or health*

### 4.  Support and Accountability

Maintain a support system that motivates you on your quest to wellness and holds you accountable. Join a healthy community or discuss your objectives with your pals.

- *Step into Action: Invite a friend or relative to join you on a wellness challenge or goal by getting in touch with them.*

## 5. Mindfulness-Based Eating

To make deliberate meal selections that nourish your body and support your health objectives, keep practicing mindful eating.

*Action Step: During each meal, practice one mindful eating technique, such as enjoying every bite or avoiding distractions.*

## 6. Stress Management
Make stress management a top priority to prevent stress from impairing your ability to control your blood sugar and general well-being.

Try out a new stress-reduction technique, such as progressive muscle relaxation or mindfulness meditation.

## 7. Celebrate Milestones

Celebrate your victories and landmarks as you progress toward a sugar-free lifestyle. Give yourself credit for your effort and advancement.

*Action Step: Plan a celebration or reward for yourself when you reach one of your long-term wellness objectives*

Your sugar cleanse has served as a foundation for a happier, healthier future. As you continue to give management of your blood sugar and your general well-being top priority, embrace the possibilities that lie ahead. Your dedication, tenacity, and willpower have contributed to your sugar-free future.

**Summary**

In this last chapter, we've celebrated your transition from reset to transformation, looked back on your successes, and looked forward to your future without sugar. Keep in mind that the road to long-term well-being is not a straight one as you proceed. There are many opportunities for growth, difficulties, and lifelong learning.

Your future of sugar control, health, and vitality is within your grasp. You're well-equipped to travel this route with assurance and grace if you set sustainable objectives, incorporate healthy habits, stay informed, seek assistance, practice mindful eating, manage stress, and celebrate your victories.

I'm happy to hear that you finished "Sugar Reset: Your 21-Day Transformation." This is just the beginning of your journey; it develops into a lifetime commitment to your health and well-being. Accept the future you have without sugar, and may it be one of strength, harmony, and lasting wellness.

# THE END

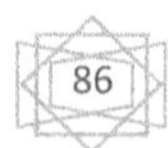

www.ingramcontent.com/pod-product-compliance
Lightning Source LLC
Chambersburg PA
CBHW050838260726
48660CB00006B/2317